Herpes Tales

Shingles, Bells Palsy, Ramsay Hunts OH NO!

Sonia Kahan MSc

4CornersTV Press

CONTENTS

Title Page

Copyright

Prologue

Disclaimer

Chapter 1: The Malevolent Mingle ... 1

Chapter 2: Shingles Strikes with Sassy Style ... 3

Chapter 3: The Quirks of Bells Palsy ... 5

Chapter 4: Ramsay Hunts: Descendant of Varicella Zoster ... 7

Chapter 5: The Herbal Avengers Take on Shingles ... 8

Chapter 6: The Herbaceous Heroes vs. Bells Palsy ... 10

Chapter 7: The Herbal Crusaders Confront Ramsay Hunt Syndrome ... 13

Chapter 8: Unveiling the Secrets of Lemon Balm ... 15

Chapter 9: Exploring the Marvels of Astragalus ... 18

Chapter 10: Unveiling the Healing Properties of St. John's Wort ... 21

Chapter 11: Unlocking the Healing Potential of Licorice ... 24

Chapter 12: Embracing the Healing Touch of Calendula ... 27

Chapter 13: Exploring the Potency of Echinacea Purpurea ... 30

Chapter 14: Ashwagandha - The Vitality Herb ... 33

Chapter 15: Unveiling the Healing Wonders of Aloe Vera ... 36

Chapter 16: The Epic Battle Against Varicella's Minions   39

Books By This Author   41

Fin   43

PROLOGUE

Post chickenpox ,VSV can show up as Shingles, Bells Palsy and Ramsay Hunts Syndrome. In this epic tale, learn the mechanisms behind each ailment and herbal remedies that can help you fight flare ups with a wealth of herbal lore and materia medica too.

DISCLAIMER

The information provided in this herbal medicine book is intended solely for educational purposes and should not be considered medical advice. The content contained herein is not intended to diagnose, treat, cure, or prevent any disease or medical condition.

Readers are strongly advised to consult with a licensed medical practitioner or healthcare professional before making any changes to their medical regimen, including the use of herbal remedies or supplements. Each individual's health circumstances are unique, and what may be safe and effective for one person may not be suitable for another.

The author, publisher, and contributors of this book are not liable for any consequences arising from the use or misuse of the information provided herein. The use of herbal remedies should be approached with caution and under the guidance of qualified medical professionals.

Furthermore, it is essential to recognize that herbal medicine is not a replacement for conventional medical treatment. It can complement traditional healthcare approaches but should not be used as a substitute without proper medical supervision.

Additionally, readers should exercise discretion and conduct their own research to verify the accuracy and reliability of the information presented in this book. While efforts have been made to ensure the accuracy of the content, no guarantee is made regarding its completeness, suitability, or applicability to any particular individual or situation.

By accessing and utilizing the information in this book, readers acknowledge and accept the inherent risks associated with using herbal remedies and agree to indemnify and hold harmless the author, publisher, and contributors from any claims, damages, or liabilities arising from such use.

In summary, always consult with a licensed medical practitioner or healthcare professional before implementing any changes to your medical regimen, and use herbal remedies responsibly and at your own risk.

CHAPTER 1: THE MALEVOLENT MINGLE

In the hidden corners of the human body, where cells whisper secrets and nerves hum with life, there dwelled a most sinister figure – Varicella Zoster, accompanied by her malevolent brood. Among them were Chickenpox, Shingles, and the mischievous duo of Bells Palsy and Ramsay Hunts. Together, they formed a quartet of viral villainy that spread havoc and mischief wherever they roamed.

Varicella Zoster, the dark matriarch, exuded an air of calculated malice as she surveyed her domain. "My dearest companions," she purred, her voice dripping with sinister charm, "the time has come for us to unleash our wickedness upon the world above. Let us show them the true extent of our power and leave them quaking in fear."

Her malevolent brood cackled in unison, their laughter echoing through the corridors of the host. With a flick of her metaphysical tendrils, Varicella Zoster set her plan into motion, each of her companions eager to play their part in the impending chaos.

Chickenpox, the rambunctious troublemaker, dashed forth with gleeful abandon, spreading his rash and fever like a contagion of chaos. "Look upon me, mortals!" he crowed, his voice a cacophony of mischief. "I am the scourge of childhood, the bane of parents everywhere. None shall escape my itchy embrace!"

Shingles, the cunning elder sibling, slinked along nerve pathways with stealthy precision, leaving a trail of blistering pain in his wake. "Fear me, fools," he hissed, his voice a whisper of torment. "For I am the shadow that haunts your dreams, the thorn in your side that refuses to relent."

Bells Palsy and Ramsay Hunts, the mischievous duo, danced a twisted tango of paralysis and pain, their antics leaving their victims with crooked smiles and drooping eyes. "Behold our handiwork," they chortled, their voices a symphony of chaos. "We are the masters of facial folly, the jesters of neurological mischief. Bow before our might!"

Together, Varicella Zoster and her malevolent brood reveled in the havoc they wrought, their laughter mingling with the cries of their unfortunate victims. For in the realm of pathogens, there were none more cunning or malevolent than they, and their legacy of viral villainy would echo through the annals of history for eternity… so they would like to think.

CHAPTER 2: SHINGLES STRIKES WITH SASSY STYLE

In the labyrinthine pathways of the human body, where nerves intertwine like vines in a jungle, there came a visitor most unwelcome – Herpes Zoster, known colloquially as Shingles. This fiendish foe emerged with all the flair of a villain making a grand entrance, ready to wreak havoc with a touch of sassy style.

As the curtains rose on this viral drama, Herpes Zoster sauntered onto the stage, clad in a cloak of blisters and a smirk of mischief. "Ah, dear host," it purred, its voice dripping with infectious charm, "prepare to be dazzled by my performance."

With a flourish, Herpes Zoster made its presence known, igniting a symphony of tingling and burning sensations along the nerve pathways. "I am no ordinary virus," it declared, its Latin name rolling off the tongue with dramatic flair. "I am Herpes Zoster, the reactivation of Varicella Zoster, here to turn your world upside down."

But Shingles was not content to merely make an entrance; oh no, it craved attention and adoration like a diva on stage. With each passing moment, its blisters erupted into a cacophony of discomfort, leaving the host in a state of bewildered agony.

"Now, my dear host," Shingles purred, its voice a velvet whisper in the wind, "allow me to share a few important tidbits of information. First and foremost, know that I am highly contagious to those who have not yet had the pleasure of encountering my predecessor, Chickenpox."

"It is imperative that you keep your distance from the uninitiated," it continued, its tone as serious as a solo in a tragic opera. "For they may fall victim to my charms and suffer the same fate as you."

Shingles paused for dramatic effect, allowing its words to sink in before delivering the final blow. "But fear not, dear host, for there are remedies to ease your suffering. Antiviral medications and pain relievers may dull the sting of my presence, though they cannot banish me entirely."

And with that, Herpes Zoster bid adieu, leaving the host to grapple with its lingering presence. For in the world of viruses, Shingles was a force to be reckoned with, combining sass and style in a performance that would leave its mark long after the final curtain fell.

CHAPTER 3: THE QUIRKS OF BELLS PALSY

A COMEDY OF NERVE AND NONSENSE

In the bustling metropolis of the human body, where neurons mingle like gossiping socialites and muscles perform their daily routines, a peculiar pair made their entrance – Bells Palsy and the villainous Shingles, known in Latin as Herpes Zoster. Their arrival brought a touch of whimsy and mischief to the otherwise orderly domain.

Bells Palsy, with its charming asymmetry and mysterious aura, sauntered onto the stage with all the grace of a debonair rogue. "Greetings, dear host," it proclaimed, its voice a melodious whisper. "Prepare to be bewitched by my peculiar brand of paralysis."

With a flick of its metaphorical wand, Bells Palsy cast its spell, leaving one side of the face drooping like a wilting flower. "Fear not, my dear," it assured, its tone as soothing as a cup of herbal tea. "For though I may distort your visage, I am but a temporary inconvenience, here to add a dash of quirkiness to your life."

Meanwhile, lurking in the shadows like a sinister specter, Shingles made its presence known with a flourish of blisters and a wicked grin. "Ah, the drama unfolds," it hissed, its voice dripping with villainy. "I am Herpes Zoster, the reactivation of Varicella Zoster, here to remind you of the perils of my predecessor, Chickenpox."

With a touch of its metaphorical claws, Shingles ignited a symphony of tingling and burning sensations along the nerve pathways. "Behold my power," it declared proudly, reveling in the chaos it unleashed. "For I am Shingles, the harbinger of discomfort and the scourge of unsuspecting hosts."

As the drama unfolded within the body's bustling theater, the host found themselves caught in a whirlwind of whimsy and villainy. Bells Palsy added its quirky charm to the performance, while Shingles brought a touch of drama and discomfort to the stage.

But fear not, dear reader, for amidst the chaos and confusion, there are lessons to be learned. For those grappling with the villainous Shingles, it is crucial to seek medical attention promptly and follow the prescribed treatment regimen to alleviate discomfort and prevent complications. And for those visited by the whimsical Bells Palsy, take heart in knowing that it is but a temporary visitor, destined to fade away like a passing breeze.

And so, as the curtain falls on this chapter of the Chronicles of Varicella, the host is left to navigate the whims and wiles of Bells Palsy and the villainous Shingles, knowing that amidst the chaos, there is always hope for everlasting relief.

CHAPTER 4: RAMSAY HUNTS: DESCENDANT OF VARICELLA ZOSTER

In the bustling metropolis of Microbia, amidst the chaos of cellular activity, a new character emerged. His name? Ramsay Hunts. But Ray wasn't your ordinary protagonist. No, he was a descendant of the infamous Varicella Zoster virus, and he had quite the reputation to uphold.

As the morning sun rose over the horizon of the host's body, Ramsay Hunts began his daily routine. With a mischievous twinkle in his molecular eyes, he set off on his quest for domination within the vast landscape of the dermal layer.

Ray was not one to be underestimated. He moved with stealth and precision, slipping past the body's defenses with ease. His infectious charm was matched only by his insatiable appetite for adventure.

But what truly set Ray apart was his unique behavior. Unlike his ancestors, who often wreaked havoc and left destruction in their wake, Ray had a different approach. He was a master of subtlety, weaving his way through the body's tissues with finesse.

CHAPTER 5: THE HERBAL AVENGERS TAKE ON SHINGLES

In the bustling town of Dermatopolis, where the streets were paved with skin cells and the air was thick with humidity, a villainous intruder had infiltrated the populace – none other than the notorious Shingles. But fear not, for when trouble rears its ugly head, the Herbal Avengers are always ready to spring into action!

Leading the charge is Lemon Balm, known by its Latin alias, Melissa officinalis. With a tangy twist and a hint of citrus charm, Lemon Balm wastes no time in unleashing its arsenal of antiviral compounds, including rosmarinic acid and flavonoids. Its mission? To thwart Shingles' nefarious plans and soothe the inflamed skin with its calming properties.

Echinacea, the stalwart defender of immune health, strides onto the scene with its Latin name, Echinacea purpurea, proudly emblazoned upon its cape. Rich in polysaccharides and alkamides, Echinacea rallies the body's defenses and helps to shorten the duration and severity of Shingles outbreaks.

Licorice, the sweet and steadfast ally of herbal medicine, charges forth with its Latin name, Glycyrrhiza glabra, gleaming like a beacon of hope in the darkness. Its active compound, glycyrrhizin, boasts potent antiviral properties that work to inhibit the replication of the Shingles virus, while its soothing effects help to calm the irritated skin.

Calendula, the Sunshine Soother, joins the fray with its Latin name, Calendula officinalis, shining brightly in the midst of battle. Rich in flavonoids and triterpenoids, Calendula's anti-inflammatory actions help to alleviate the pain and discomfort caused by Shingles' blistering rash, while promoting healing and regeneration of the affected tissues.

St. John's Wort, the radiant defender of nerve pain relief, makes its presence known with its Latin name, Hypericum perforatum, blazing like a beacon of hope amidst the chaos. Its active constituents, hypericin and hyperforin, work to alleviate the nerve pain and tingling sensations that often accompany Shingles outbreaks, providing much-needed relief to the afflicted.

Last but certainly not least, Aloe Vera emerges as the cool-headed healer of the group, its Latin name, Aloe barbadensis, shimmering with soothing potential. With its polysaccharides and anthraquinones, Aloe Vera provides instant relief to the burning and itching sensations caused by Shingles, while promoting healing and regeneration of the damaged skin.

Together, the Herbaceous Heroes stand united against Shingles, their combined forces proving too formidable for the viral menace to withstand. With a flourish of botanical brilliance, they vanquish the foe and restore peace and tranquility to the skin of Dermatopolis once more.

And so, as the sun sets on the horizon, the citizens of Dermatopolis rejoice, grateful for the unwavering courage and herbal heroics of their beloved Herbaceous Heroes. For in the face of adversity, it is the healing power of nature's finest defenders that reigns supreme, proving that even the most formidable foes can be conquered with a little help from Mother Earth's green guardians.

CHAPTER 6: THE HERBACEOUS HEROES VS. BELLS PALSY

In the quaint hamlet of Nervana, nestled snugly within the neural pathways, a sinister foe had set its sights on wreaking havoc – none other than the dreaded Bells Palsy. But fear not, for when trouble brews, the Herbaceous Heroes are always ready to spring into action!

Leading the charge is Lemon Balm, known by its Latin moniker, Melissa officinalis. With a zesty demeanor and a tangy twist, Lemon Balm unleashes its potent antiviral constituents, including rosmarinic acid and flavonoids. Its mission? To thwart Bells Palsy's mischievous machinations and restore balance to the facial nerves.

Skullcap, the serene sentinel of nervous system health, strides forth with determination. Its Latin name, Scutellaria lateriflora, graces its cape as it dives headfirst into battle. Skullcap's soothing actions, fueled by its potent flavonoids and alkaloids, work to calm the spasms and twitching often associated with Bells Palsy's unwelcome visit.

Ashwagandha, the mighty adaptogen, joins the fray with its Latin name, Withania somnifera, proudly displayed. Its constituents, including with anolides and alkaloids, bolster the body's resilience and combat the stress and inflammation triggered by Bells Palsy's assault.

Licorice, the sweet and steadfast ally of herbal medicine, strides confidently onto the battlefield with its Latin name, Glycyrrhiza glabra, emblazoned upon its shield. Its anti-inflammatory compounds, such as glycyrrhizin and flavonoids, work tirelessly to reduce swelling and promote healing in the affected facial nerves.

Ginkgo Biloba, the wise and venerable sage of herbal lore, lends its support to the cause with its Latin name, Ginkgo biloba, leading the charge. Rich in flavonoids and terpenoids, Ginkgo Biloba enhances circulation and oxygenation to the brain, aiding in the recovery of nerve function compromised by Bells Palsy's relentless onslaught.

Turmeric, the golden goddess of anti-inflammatory prowess, steps onto the battlefield with its Latin name, Curcuma longa, gleaming brightly. Its active compound, curcumin, launches a full-scale assault against inflammation and oxidative stress, offering relief to the tissues besieged by Bells Palsy's relentless assault.

Last but certainly not least, St. John's Wort, the radiant defender of nerve pain relief, makes its presence known with its Latin name, Hypericum perforatum, shining like a beacon of hope in the darkness. Its constituents, including hypericin and hyperforin, soothe the discomfort and tingling sensations that often accompany Bells Palsy's unwelcome intrusion.

Together, the Herbaceous Heroes stand united against Bells Palsy, their combined forces proving too formidable for the villainous affliction to withstand. With a flourish of herbal heroics, they vanquish the foe and restore peace and tranquility to the neural pathways of Nervana once more.

And so, as the sun sets on the horizon, the citizens of Nervana rejoice, grateful for the unwavering courage and botanical brilliance of their beloved Herbaceous Heroes. For in the face of adversity, it is the healing power of nature's finest defenders that reigns supreme, proving that even the most daunting challenges can be overcome with a little help from Mother Earth's green guardians.

CHAPTER 7: THE HERBAL CRUSADERS CONFRONT RAMSAY HUNT SYNDROME

In the bustling town of Neuroville, where nerve signals crackled like fireworks on a summer night, a villainous intruder had infiltrated the community – Ramsay Hunt Syndrome. But fear not, for when trouble arises, the Herbal Crusaders are always ready to spring into action!

Leading the charge is Lemon Balm, known by its Latin alias, Melissa officinalis. With a zesty flair and a hint of citrus charm, Lemon Balm unleashes its potent antiviral compounds, including rosmarinic acid and flavonoids. Its mission? To thwart Ramsay Hunt Syndrome's dastardly plans and provide relief from the painful blisters and facial paralysis it inflicts.

Echinacea, the valiant guardian of immune health, strides onto the scene with its Latin name, Echinacea purpurea, proudly emblazoned upon its shield. Rich in polysaccharides and alkamides, Echinacea rallies the body's defenses and helps to shorten the duration and severity of Ramsay Hunt Syndrome outbreaks.

Licorice, the sweet and steadfast ally of herbal medicine, charges forth with its Latin name, Glycyrrhiza glabra, gleaming like a beacon of hope in the darkness. Its active compound, glycyrrhizin, boasts potent antiviral properties that work to inhibit the replication of the Ramsay Hunt Syndrome virus, while its soothing effects help to calm the inflamed nerves and reduce pain.

Astragalus, the resilient root renowned for its immune-boosting prowess, joins the fray with its Latin name, Astragalus membranaceus, blazing with vitality. Its polysaccharides and flavonoids bolster the body's defenses, helping to combat the viral infection and promote nerve regeneration in those affected by Ramsay Hunt Syndrome.

Together, the Herbal Crusaders stand united against Ramsay Hunt Syndrome, their combined forces proving too formidable for the viral menace to withstand. With a flourish of botanical brilliance, they vanquish the foe and restore hope and vitality to the people of Neuroville once more.

And so, as the sun sets on the horizon, the citizens of Neuroville rejoice, grateful for the unwavering courage and herbal heroics of their beloved Herbal Crusaders. For in the face of adversity, it is the healing power of nature's finest defenders that reigns supreme, proving that even the most formidable foes can be conquered with a little help from Mother Earth's green guardians.

CHAPTER 8: UNVEILING THE SECRETS OF LEMON BALM

In the verdant gardens of herbal lore, Lemon Balm reigns supreme, offering its gentle embrace to those in need of solace and healing. Let us embark on a journey to uncover the treasures hidden within this remarkable herb.

Latin Name: Melissa officinalis

Constituents:
- Essential oils (including citral, citronellal, and geraniol)
- Flavonoids (such as quercetin and luteolin)
- Rosmarinic acid
- Tannins
- Polyphenols

Actions:
1. **Calming:** Lemon Balm is renowned for its soothing properties, helping to ease anxiety, stress, and nervous tension.
2. **Antiviral:** It exhibits antiviral activity, making it useful in fighting off cold sores, herpes outbreaks, and other viral infections.
3. **Antioxidant:** Lemon Balm's high antioxidant content helps to protect cells from damage caused by free radicals.
4. **Digestive:** It aids digestion and can alleviate symptoms of indigestion, bloating, and gas.
5. **Sleep Aid**: Lemon Balm promotes relaxation and can improve sleep quality, making it ideal for those struggling with insomnia.

Cautions:

- Lemon Balm is generally considered safe for most people when used in moderation. However, some individuals may experience mild side effects such as stomach upset or allergic reactions.

- If you are pregnant, nursing, or have a pre-existing medical condition, it's best to consult with a healthcare professional before using Lemon Balm therapeutically.

- Lemon Balm may interact with certain medications, particularly sedatives and thyroid medications. If you are taking any prescription medications, speak with your doctor before incorporating Lemon Balm into your routine.

Easy Recipes:

1. Lemon Balm Tea:
   - Ingredients:
     - 1 tablespoon fresh lemon balm leaves (or 1 teaspoon dried)
     - 1 cup boiling water
   - Instructions:
     1. Place the lemon balm leaves in a mug.
     2. Pour boiling water over the leaves.
     3. Cover and steep for 5-10 minutes. AND NO LONGER
     4. Strain and sweeten with honey, if desired. Enjoy this soothing tea before bed or during moments of stress.

2. Lemon Balm Infused Oil:
   - Ingredients:
     - 1 cup fresh lemon balm leaves (washed and dried)
     - 1 cup carrier oil (such as olive oil or almond oil)
   - Instructions:
     1. Place the lemon balm leaves in a clean, dry glass jar.
     2. Pour the carrier oil over the leaves, ensuring they are fully submerged.
     3. Seal the jar tightly and place it in a sunny spot for 2-4 weeks to infuse.
     4. Strain out the lemon balm leaves and transfer the infused oil to a clean glass bottle for storage.
     5. Use this aromatic Lemon Balm-infused oil as a massage

oil, moisturizer, or as a base for homemade salves and balms.

With these simple recipes and precautions in mind, you can harness the healing power of Lemon Balm to enhance your well-being and nourish your body and soul. Whether sipping on a comforting cup of tea or indulging in a relaxing massage, let Lemon Balm be your guide to tranquility and vitality.

CHAPTER 9: EXPLORING THE MARVELS OF ASTRAGALUS

Step into the world of Astragalus, an ancient herb revered for its immune-boosting properties and remarkable healing potential. Join me as we uncover the secrets of this extraordinary plant and discover how it can nourish and fortify the body from within.

Latin Name: Astragalus membranaceus

Constituents:
- Polysaccharides (including astragalans and arabinogalactans)
- Saponins (such as astragalosides)
- Flavonoids
- Amino acids
- Trace minerals (including zinc, selenium, and iron)

Actions:
1. **Immune Support**: Astragalus is renowned for its ability to strengthen the immune system, making it a valuable ally during times of illness or when facing immune challenges.
2. **Adaptogenic:** It helps the body adapt to stress and promotes overall resilience and vitality.
3. **Anti-inflammatory:** Astragalus exhibits anti-inflammatory properties, which can help reduce inflammation and promote healing throughout the body.
4. **Cardioprotective:** It supports cardiovascular health by improving circulation, lowering blood pressure, and reducing cholesterol levels.
5. **Antioxidant:** Astragalus is rich in antioxidants, which help

protect cells from damage caused by free radicals and oxidative stress.

Cautions:

- While Astragalus is generally considered safe for most people when used appropriately, it may interact with certain medications, including immunosuppressants and blood thinners. If you are taking any prescription medications, consult with your healthcare provider before using Astragalus.

- Pregnant and breastfeeding women should also exercise caution and consult with a healthcare professional before using Astragalus.

Easy Recipes:

1. Astragalus Immune-Boosting Tea:
   - Ingredients:
     - 1 tablespoon dried Astragalus root slices
     - 2 cups water
     - Optional: honey or lemon to taste
   - Instructions:
     1. In a small saucepan, add water and dried astragalus root.
     2. Bring the water to boil.
     3. Reduce heat to low, cover, and simmer for 20-30 minutes.
     4. Remove from heat and let the tea steep for an additional 10 minutes.
     5. Strain the tea and discard the Astragalus root slices.
     6. Add honey or lemon to taste, if desired. Enjoy this immune-boosting tea daily to support overall health and vitality.

2. Astragalus Root Tincture:
   - Ingredients:
     - 1 part dried Astragalus root (chopped or powdered)
     - 2 parts alcohol (such as vodka or brandy)
   - Instructions:
     1. Place the dried Astragalus root in a clean glass jar.
     2. Pour the alcohol over the Astragalus root, ensuring it is

completely submerged.

    3. Place wax paper on top and seal the jar tightly and shake well to combine.

    4. Store the jar in a cool, dark place for 4-6 weeks, shaking it occasionally.

    5. After the tincture has finished macerating, strain it through a fine mesh strainer or cheesecloth into a clean glass bottle.

    6. Label the bottle with the date and contents. Take 1-2 dropperfuls (approximately 30-60 drops) of the tincture daily to support immune health and overall well-being.

With these simple recipes and cautions in mind, you can unlock the immune-boosting power of Astragalus and nourish your body from the inside out. Whether sipping on a comforting cup of tea or incorporating a tincture into your daily routine, let Astragalus be your ally in achieving optimal health and vitality.

CHAPTER 10: UNVEILING THE HEALING PROPERTIES OF ST. JOHN'S WORT

Step into the world of St. John's Wort, a bright and cheerful herb that has been cherished for centuries for its healing properties and sunny disposition. Join me as we explore the depths of its medicinal virtues and learn how to harness its power for health and well-being.

Latin Name: Hypericum perforatum

Constituents:
- Hypericin
- Hyperforin
- Flavonoids (including quercetin and rutin)
- Tannins
- Essential oils

Actions:

1. **Antidepressant:** St. John's Wort is best known for its antidepressant properties, making it a popular natural remedy for mild to moderate depression and anxiety.

2. **Anti-inflammatory:** It exhibits anti-inflammatory effects, which can help reduce pain and inflammation throughout the body.

3. **Antiviral:** St. John's Wort has antiviral properties and may be effective against certain viruses, including the herpes simplex virus.

4. **Nervine:** It acts as a nervine tonic, helping to calm the nervous system and promote relaxation.

5. **Wound Healing**: St. John's Wort has a long history of use in promoting wound healing and reducing scarring when applied topically.

Cautions:

- St. John's Wort may interact with certain medications, including antidepressants, birth control pills, and blood thinners. If you are taking any prescription medications, consult with your healthcare provider before using St. John's Wort.

- It may cause photosensitivity in some individuals, making the skin more sensitive to sunlight. Avoid excessive sun exposure while using St. John's Wort, and use sunscreen or protective clothing when outdoors.

Easy Recipes:

1. **St. John's Wort Infused Oil:**
   - Ingredients:
      - 1 cup fresh St. John's Wort flowers and leaves
      - 1 cup carrier oil (such as olive oil or almond oil)
   - Instructions:

   1. Wash and dry the St. John's Wort flowers and leaves thoroughly.

   2. Place the herbs in a clean, dry glass jar.

   3. Pour the carrier oil over the herbs, ensuring they are fully submerged.

   4. Seal the jar tightly and place it in a sunny spot for 2-4 weeks to infuse.

   5. Strain out the herbs and transfer the infused oil to a clean glass bottle for storage.

   6. Use this aromatic St. John's Wort-infused oil topically to soothe minor burns, bruises, and wounds.

2. St. John's Wort Tea:
   - Ingredients:

- 1 tablespoon dried St. John's Wort flowers and leaves

- 1 cup boiling water

- Instructions:

1. Place the dried St. John's Wort flowers and leaves in a teapot or mug.

2. Pour boiling water over the herbs.

3. Cover and steep for 5-10 minutes.

4. Strain and sweeten with honey, if desired. Enjoy this calming tea to uplift the spirits and promote relaxation.

With these simple recipes and cautions in mind, you can harness the healing power of St. John's Wort to support your mental and physical well-being. Whether applying a soothing infused oil to your skin or sipping on a comforting cup of tea, let St. John's Wort be your ally in achieving optimal health and vitality.

CHAPTER 11: UNLOCKING THE HEALING POTENTIAL OF LICORICE

Welcome to the world of Licorice, a sweet and soothing herb that has been cherished for centuries for its medicinal properties and delectable flavor. Join me as we delve into the depths of its healing virtues and discover how to incorporate this remarkable herb into your daily routine.

Latin Name: Glycyrrhiza glabra

Constituents:
- Glycyrrhizin
- Flavonoids (including liquiritin and glabridin)
- Saponins
- Coumarins
- Polysaccharides

Actions:
1. Demulcent: Licorice acts as a demulcent, forming a protective coating over mucous membranes to soothe and protect irritated tissues.

2. Expectorant: It helps to loosen and expel mucus from the respiratory tract, making it useful for relieving coughs and congestion.

3. Anti-inflammatory: Licorice exhibits anti-inflammatory effects, which can help reduce inflammation and alleviate pain throughout the body.

4. Antiviral: It has antiviral properties and may be effective against certain viruses, including the herpes simplex virus.

5. Adrenal Support: Licorice supports adrenal function and can help regulate cortisol levels, making it beneficial for managing stress and fatigue.

Cautions:

- Licorice contains glycyrrhizin, which can cause mineralocorticoid excess and lead to hypertension, edema, and electrolyte imbalances in susceptible individuals. Long-term or excessive use of licorice should be avoided, especially by those with hypertension, heart disease, or kidney disorders.

- Pregnant and breastfeeding women should exercise caution when using licorice, as it may affect hormone levels and lead to complications.

Licorice root, derived from the Glycyrrhiza glabra plant, is considered rare in certain contexts due to several factors:

1. Growing Conditions: Licorice plants require specific growing conditions, including well-drained soil, plenty of sunlight, and a warm climate. They are primarily cultivated in regions such as Asia, the Mediterranean, and parts of the Middle East. Limited availability of suitable growing environments contributes to the relative rarity of licorice.

2. Slow Growth Rate: Licorice plants have a slow growth rate and can take several years to mature before they are ready for harvest. It typically takes three to five years or more for licorice roots to develop fully. This slow growth rate, coupled with high demand, contributes to the limited availability of licorice in the market.

3. High Demand: Licorice root is in high demand for its culinary and medicinal uses. It is commonly used as a flavoring agent in confectionery, beverages, and tobacco products, as well as in traditional herbal medicine. The combination of limited growing conditions and high demand contributes to the rarity of licorice.

Licorice should be used with caution due to its potential side effects and interactions with medications. Here are a few reasons why:

1. Glycyrrhizin Content: Licorice root contains a compound called glycyrrhizin, which can cause elevated blood pressure, fluid retention, and potassium loss when consumed in large amounts or over an extended period. These effects can be particularly problematic for individuals with high blood pressure, heart disease, or kidney disorders.

2. Interactions with Medications: Licorice root may interact with certain medications, including corticosteroids, diuretics, and medications for high blood pressure, diabetes, and heart conditions. It can affect the metabolism and effectiveness of these medications, leading to potential complications.

3. Pregnancy and Nursing: Licorice should be avoided during pregnancy and breastfeeding due to the risk of adverse effects on fetal development and milk production. Glycyrrhizin can cross the placenta and be excreted in breast milk, potentially affecting the developing fetus or newborn.

4. Individual Sensitivity: Some individuals may be more sensitive to the effects of licorice than others, experiencing symptoms such as headaches, fatigue, and muscle weakness with even moderate consumption.

While licorice can be enjoyed safely in moderation as part of a balanced diet or used therapeutically under the guidance of a qualified healthcare professional, it's essential to be aware of its potential risks and exercise caution, especially for individuals with underlying health conditions or those taking medications.

CHAPTER 12: EMBRACING THE HEALING TOUCH OF CALENDULA

Step into the world of Calendula, a vibrant and versatile herb that has been treasured for centuries for its therapeutic properties and radiant beauty. Join me as we explore the depths of its healing virtues and learn how to incorporate this remarkable herb into our daily lives.

Latin Name: Calendula officinalis

Constituents:
- Flavonoids (including quercetin and rutin)
- Triterpenoids
- Carotenoids (including lutein and beta-carotene)
- Saponins
- Essential oils

Actions:
1. **Anti-inflammatory:** Calendula exhibits potent anti-inflammatory effects, making it beneficial for relieving pain, swelling, and inflammation associated with various conditions.

2. **Antimicrobial:** It has antimicrobial properties, which can help inhibit the growth of bacteria and fungi, making it useful for treating minor wounds, cuts, and infections.

3. **Wound Healing:** Calendula promotes wound healing and tissue regeneration, accelerating the healing process and reducing the risk of scarring.

4. **Skin Soothing**: It soothes and moisturizes the skin, making it ideal for relieving dryness, itching, and irritation caused by eczema, dermatitis, and other skin conditions.

5. **Antioxidant:** Calendula is rich in antioxidants, which help protect cells from damage caused by free radicals and oxidative stress.

Cautions:

- While Calendula is generally considered safe for external use, some individuals may experience allergic reactions or skin irritation. Perform a patch test before using Calendula topically, especially if you have sensitive skin.

- Avoid internal use of Calendula during pregnancy and breastfeeding, as its safety has not been established for these populations.

Easy Recipes:

1. **Calendula Infused Oil:**
    - Ingredients:
      - 1 cup dried calendula flowers
      - 1 cup carrier oil (such as olive oil or almond oil)
    - Instructions:
      1. Place the dried calendula flowers in a clean, dry glass jar.
      2. Pour the carrier oil over the flowers, ensuring they are fully submerged.
      3. Seal the jar tightly and place it in a sunny spot for 2-4 weeks to infuse.
      4. Strain out the flowers and transfer the infused oil to a clean glass bottle for storage.
      5. Use this soothing Calendula-infused oil topically to relieve dry skin, soothe irritation, and promote wound healing.

2. **Calendula Salve:**
    - Ingredients:
      - ½ cup Calendula-infused oil
      - 2 tablespoons beeswax pellets

- Optional: 10-15 drops of lavender essential oil (for added fragrance and skin-soothing properties)

- Instructions:

1. In a double boiler or heat-safe bowl, combine the Calendula-infused oil and beeswax pellets.

2. Heat gently over low heat until the beeswax melts completely, stirring occasionally.

3. Remove from heat and add the optional lavender essential oil, if desired.

4. Pour the mixture into clean, sterilized jars or tins and allow it to cool and solidify before sealing.

5. Use this nourishing Calendula salve topically to soothe dry, irritated skin, promote wound healing, and protect against environmental damage.

With these simple recipes and cautions in mind, you can harness the healing power of Calendula to nurture and protect your skin, body, and soul. Whether infusing oil for topical use or creating a soothing salve, let Calendula be your ally in achieving radiant health and well-being.

CHAPTER 13: EXPLORING THE POTENCY OF ECHINACEA PURPUREA

Welcome to the realm of Echinacea Purpurea, a formidable herb celebrated for its immune-boosting prowess and therapeutic benefits. Join me as we embark on a journey to uncover the secrets of this remarkable plant and learn how to harness its power for optimal health and vitality.

Latin Name: Echinacea purpurea

Constituents:
- Alkamides (including echinacein and echinacoside)
- Polysaccharides
- Flavonoids
- Essential oils
- Glycoproteins

Actions:
1. **Immune Support:** Echinacea Purpurea is renowned for its ability to strengthen the immune system, making it a valuable ally during times of illness or when facing immune challenges.

2. **Anti-inflammatory:** It exhibits anti-inflammatory effects, which can help reduce inflammation and alleviate symptoms associated with conditions such as colds, flu, and respiratory infections.

3. **Antiviral:** Echinacea Purpurea has antiviral properties and may be effective against certain viruses, including the common

cold and influenza viruses.

4. **Antioxidant:** It is rich in antioxidants, which help protect cells from damage caused by free radicals and oxidative stress.

5. **Wound Healing:** Echinacea Purpurea promotes wound healing and tissue regeneration, accelerating the healing process and reducing the risk of infection.

Cautions:

- While Echinacea Purpurea is generally considered safe for most people when used appropriately, some individuals may experience allergic reactions or gastrointestinal upset. If you have a known allergy to plants in the Asteraceae family (such as ragweed, marigolds, or daisies), use Echinacea with caution.

- Avoid long-term or excessive use of Echinacea Purpurea, as this may lead to decreased effectiveness over time and potential side effects.

- Pregnant and breastfeeding women should consult with a healthcare professional before using Echinacea Purpurea, as its safety has not been established for these populations.

Easy Recipes:

1. Echinacea Purpurea Tea:
   - Ingredients:
      - 1 teaspoon dried Echinacea Purpurea root or aerial parts
      - 1 cup boiling water
   - Instructions:

1. Place the dried Echinacea Purpurea in a teapot with water.

2. Bring the water to a boil.

3. Cover and steep for 15-20 minutes.

4. Strain and sweeten with honey or lemon, if desired. Enjoy this immune-boosting tea daily to support overall health and vitality.

2. Echinacea Purpurea Tincture:
   - Ingredients:

- 1 part dried Echinacea Purpurea root or aerial parts

- 2 parts alcohol (such as vodka or brandy)

- Instructions:

1. Place the dried Echinacea Purpurea in a clean glass jar.

2. Pour the alcohol over the herb, ensuring it is fully submerged.

3. Seal the jar tightly and shake well to combine.

4. Store the jar in a cool, dark place for 4-6 weeks, shaking it occasionally.

5. After the tincture has finished macerating, strain it through a fine mesh strainer or cheesecloth into a clean glass bottle.

6. Label the bottle with the date and contents. Take 1-2 dropperfuls (approximately 30-60 drops) of the tincture daily to support immune health and overall well-being.

With these simple recipes and cautions in mind, you can harness the immune-boosting power of Echinacea Purpurea to strengthen your defenses and promote optimal health and vitality. Whether sipping on a comforting cup of tea or incorporating a tincture into your daily routine, let Echinacea Purpurea be your ally in achieving radiant health and well-being.

CHAPTER 14: ASHWAGANDHA - THE VITALITY HERB

Introduction to Ashwagandha:

Ashwagandha (Withania somnifera), also known as Indian ginseng or winter cherry, is a revered herb in Ayurvedic medicine for its adaptogenic properties. Adaptogens are substances that help the body adapt to stressors, promoting balance and resilience. Ashwagandha has been used for centuries to support overall health and well-being, enhance vitality, and improve resilience to stress.

Materia Medica:

- Constituents: Ashwagandha contains a variety of bioactive compounds, including alkaloids, steroidal lactones (withanolides), saponins, and phenolic compounds. These constituents contribute to its pharmacological effects, including anti-stress, anti-inflammatory, antioxidant, immunomodulatory, and neuroprotective properties.

- **Actions:**

- **Adaptogenic:** Helps the body adapt to stress and maintain balance.

- **Anxiolytic:** Reduces anxiety and promotes relaxation.

- **Immunomodulatory:** Modulates immune function, supporting overall health.

- **Anti-inflammatory:** Reduces inflammation and associated symptoms.

- **Antioxidant:** Protects against oxidative stress and cellular damage.

- **Uses:**
  - Stress management
  - Anxiety and mood support
  - Immune support
  - Cognitive function and memory enhancement
  - Physical endurance and stamina
  - Sexual health and libido enhancement

Caution:

- Ashwagandha is generally considered safe for most people when used as directed. However, it may interact with certain medications or medical conditions. Consult with a healthcare professional before using ashwagandha, especially if you are pregnant, breastfeeding, have a medical condition, or are taking medications.

Recipes:

1. Ashwagandha Chai Latte:
  - Ingredients:
    - 1 cup milk (dairy or plant-based)
    - 1 teaspoon ashwagandha powder
    - 1 teaspoon chai spice blend (or cinnamon, cardamom, ginger)
    - 1 teaspoon honey or maple syrup (optional)
  - Instructions:
    1. In a small saucepan, heat the milk over medium heat until hot but not boiling.
    2. Whisk in the ashwagandha powder and chai spice blend until well combined.
    3. Remove from heat and sweeten with honey or maple syrup if desired.
    4. Pour into a mug and enjoy as a soothing and nourishing beverage.

2. Ashwagandha Energy Balls:
  - Ingredients:

- 1 cup rolled oats
- 1/2 cup nut butter (such as almond or peanut butter)
- 1/4 cup honey or maple syrup
- 2 tablespoons ashwagandha powder
- 1/4 cup chopped nuts or seeds (such as almonds, walnuts, or pumpkin seeds)
- 1/4 cup dried fruit (such as raisins, dates, or cranberries)
- Optional add-ins: chocolate chips, shredded coconut, vanilla extract
- Instructions:

1. In a large mixing bowl, combine the rolled oats, nut butter, honey or maple syrup, and ashwagandha powder.

2. Mix until well combined, then fold in the chopped nuts or seeds and dried fruit.

3. Optional: Add any additional add-ins of your choice, such as chocolate chips or shredded coconut.

4. Roll the mixture into small balls using your hands, then place them on a baking sheet lined with parchment paper.

5. Refrigerate the energy balls for at least 30 minutes to firm up before serving.

6. Enjoy as a nutritious and energizing snack on-the-go.

Conclusion:

Ashwagandha is a versatile herb with a wide range of health benefits, from stress management to immune support. Incorporating ashwagandha into your wellness routine through recipes like the Ashwagandha Chai Latte and Ashwagandha Energy Balls can be a delicious and convenient way to harness its healing properties. However, remember to use ashwagandha with caution and consult with a healthcare professional if you have any concerns or underlying health conditions.

CHAPTER 15: UNVEILING THE HEALING WONDERS OF ALOE VERA

Step into the world of Aloe Vera, a succulent plant revered for its soothing properties and versatile healing abilities. Join me as we explore the depths of its medicinal virtues and learn how to harness its power for health and wellness.

Latin Name: Aloe vera

Constituents:
- Polysaccharides (including acemannan)
- Anthraquinones (such as aloin and emodin)
- Enzymes (including amylase and lipase)
- Vitamins (including vitamins A, C, and E)
- Minerals (such as calcium, magnesium, and zinc)

Actions:
1. **Skin Healing**: Aloe Vera is renowned for its ability to promote wound healing and soothe skin irritations, burns, and sunburns. Its cooling and moisturizing properties make it an ideal remedy for various skin conditions, including eczema, psoriasis, and acne.

2. **Anti-inflammatory:** It exhibits anti-inflammatory effects, which can help reduce inflammation and alleviate pain associated with conditions such as arthritis, rheumatism, and inflammatory skin conditions.

3. **Digestive Support:** Aloe Vera aids digestion and can help alleviate symptoms of indigestion, bloating, and constipation. Its

mild laxative effects help promote bowel regularity and relieve occasional constipation.

4. **Immune Support**: It supports immune health and may help the body fight off infections and viruses due to its antiviral and antibacterial properties.

5. **Hydration:** Aloe Vera is rich in water and helps hydrate the body, making it beneficial for maintaining healthy skin, hair, and overall hydration levels.

Cautions:

- While Aloe Vera is generally safe for topical use, some individuals may experience allergic reactions or skin irritation. Perform a patch test before using Aloe Vera topically, especially if you have sensitive skin.

- Avoid ingesting Aloe Vera latex, as it contains anthraquinones that can have laxative effects and may cause abdominal cramps, diarrhea, and electrolyte imbalances.

- Pregnant and breastfeeding women should consult with a healthcare professional before using Aloe Vera internally or externally, as its safety has not been established for these populations.

Easy Recipes:

1. **Aloe Vera Gel:**
   - Ingredients:
     - 1 fresh Aloe Vera leaf
   - Instructions:

   1. Wash the Aloe Vera leaf thoroughly under running water to remove any dirt or debris.

   2. Using a sharp knife, carefully slice off the serrated edges of the leaf and cut open lengthwise to expose the gel inside.

   3. Scoop out the gel with a spoon and transfer it to a clean container.

   4. Store the Aloe Vera gel in the refrigerator for up to one week. Apply the gel topically to soothe sunburns, skin irritations, and other skin conditions.

2. **Aloe Vera Juice:**
   - Ingredients:
      - 1 fresh Aloe Vera leaf
      - Optional: lemon juice, honey, or fruit juice for flavor
   - Instructions:
      1. Wash the Aloe Vera leaf thoroughly under running water.
      2. Using a sharp knife, carefully remove the thorny edges of the leaf and cut it into small pieces.
      3. Place the Aloe Vera pieces in a blender and blend until smooth.
      4. Strain the mixture through a fine mesh strainer or cheesecloth to remove any pulp or debris.
      5. Add optional flavorings such as lemon juice, honey, or fruit juice to taste.
      6. Store the Aloe Vera juice in the refrigerator and consume within 3-4 days. Drink 1-2 ounces daily for digestive support and hydration.

With these simple recipes and cautions in mind, you can harness the healing power of Aloe Vera to support your skin, digestion, and overall well-being. Whether applying soothing gel to your skin or sipping on refreshing juice, let Aloe Vera be your ally in achieving radiant health and vitality.

CHAPTER 16: THE EPIC BATTLE AGAINST VARICELLA'S MINIONS

In the tumultuous realm of health and wellness, a formidable alliance has formed—a league of extraordinary herbs ready to wage war against the nefarious minions of Varicella Zoster. Lemon Balm, Ashwagandha, Licorice, Aloe Vera, Echinacea, St. John's Wort, and Astragalus have joined forces, wielding their potent powers in a valiant effort to vanquish Shingles, Bells Palsy, and Ramsay Hunt Syndrome.

Picture it: Lemon Balm, the calming commander-in-chief, leading the charge with its soothing touch and antiviral might. Ashwagandha, the adaptogenic warrior, bolstering resilience and fortitude in the face of adversity. Licorice, the sweet strategist, marshaling its anti-inflammatory forces to quell the flames of inflammation.

But let us not forget Aloe Vera, the hydrating healer, soothing burns and wounds with its gentle touch. Echinacea, the immune-boosting sentinel, standing guard against invading pathogens with its formidable defenses. St. John's Wort, the mood-lifting champion, banishing the shadows of despair with its sunny disposition.

And then there's Astragalus, the stalwart guardian, fortifying the troops and bolstering their immune defenses with its potent arsenal of polysaccharides and antioxidants. Together, they form an unstoppable force, a united front against the relentless onslaught of Varicella's minions.

Yet, even as they celebrate their victories, our intrepid heroes know that the war is far from over. For every battle won, new challenges arise, and the fight against Shingles, Bells Palsy, and Ramsay Hunt Syndrome rages on. But with Lemon Balm, Ashwagandha, Licorice, Aloe Vera, Echinacea, St. John's Wort, and Astragalus leading the charge, there is hope on the horizon.

So, dear reader, take heart and heed the call to arms. Arm yourself with the healing power of nature's bounty, and together, we shall prevail against Varicella's minions, one battle at a time.

BOOKS BY THIS AUTHOR

Had Chickenpox, How's The Herpes?

Hurry up and get over it. Remember this? The train of thought which ravaged households all across the West in the 1980's, caused many unknowing individuals to be plagued with a lifelong enemy, herpes. The idea of having multiple days off of school, eating ice cream and watching tv in bed, yep thought we were rocking it, well varicella rocked us.

Herpes Tales: Herbal Guardians Unite!

Are you into adventure? Do you want to know how it goes down on those tough internal streets? Well here is a book for you. Journey with us as we see what happens when theraputic herbs come to the aid of human beings.

FIN